LOSING WEIGHT

It Is *Sooo* Easy

A man's simple journey to losing weight

Frank Cachia

A Catalogue-in-Publication is available from the National Library of Australia.

ISBN: 978-0-9946154-4-2

1st Edition

Acknowledgement

A special thanks to my physiotherapist for his advice and patience, when it came to proof reading.

Foreword

I came to know Frank after he had requested a referral to a dietitian from his local GP to assist him with his weight loss journey. At our initial consultation, Frank expressed his desperation to reduce his weight, clearly frustrated at his failure to lose weight after trialling a number of diets with no substantial results. He also expressed his confusion and boredom of the restricted foods he was consuming.

Frank's story portrays his understanding of how to achieve sustainable weight loss, in his own words, which comes from realigning his thoughts and approaches to food through a deeper interest to learn, ask questions and implement information around food choices. As a dietitian, this empowerment in individuals is what we aim to give and so it has been a wonderful experience to see Frank widen his perspective on food, and realizing the importance of enjoyment and balance for long term success.

Although Frank faces many challenges, including his limited ability to exercise, Frank's determination has been the most outstanding and consistent attribute I've noticed and he continues to teach me that sometimes people can go beyond what we think they're capable of and to never set the bar too low.

Carla Johnson, BND
Accredited Practising Dietitian
Melbourne
June 2017

KILSYTH MEDICAL GROUP
P.O. Box 188, Kilsyth, Victoria 3137
Ph: (03) 9725 5444   Fax: (03) 9723 5265

Dr. Harbans Gupta
MBBS, FRACGP, FAMAS
Provider No. 051732H

Dr. Chris Mason
MBChB (UK), MRCGP, FRACGP
Provider No. 2131088H

Dr. Paul Cartwright
MBBS, Cert. Aviation Med.
Dip. Hypno, Dip. Acupunc.
Provider No. 470372W

Dr. Inam Khan
MBBS, FRACGP
Provider No. 239815YA

This is the layman's guide to successful weight loss- it is exquisitely simple.

There are no drugs, potions nor mumbo jumbo; there is no crazy exercise program, no faddish diet, no psychologist to understand why you're fat.

Just plain common-sense.

Enjoy the old you in a smaller you.

I recommend this mini Bible to everyone.

Dr. Paul Cartwright
Kilsyth Medical Group

Contents

Introduction

Hello, there's absolutely nothing special about me. I suffer from aches and pains just like you. If it wasn't for the fact that sometimes I show a gregarious nature, I'm just a quiet unassuming old man.

Over an unspecified time period, I successfully changed my lifestyle and lost weight until I reached and passed my nominated weight limit without breaking a sweat. I did it so easily, so effortlessly that I want to tell you about it.

Why, because I strongly believe that by following the way I did it, it will help you lose weight and reach your desired goal!

The Reason

There are numerous reasons why people want to lose weight. In my case, it's because I simply started having trouble fitting into most of my clothing.

This came about because in April 2007 I was involved in a rather horrific industrial accident, resulting in a severely damaged left leg. An active lifestyle literally came to an abrupt end. During and after four operations and 44 months, I walked around with the aid of two crutches. Three weeks after I successful walked without the crutches, I was involved in a road accident, again badly damaging the same leg. Three more operations and another 14 months were to pass before I was again able to walk unaided.

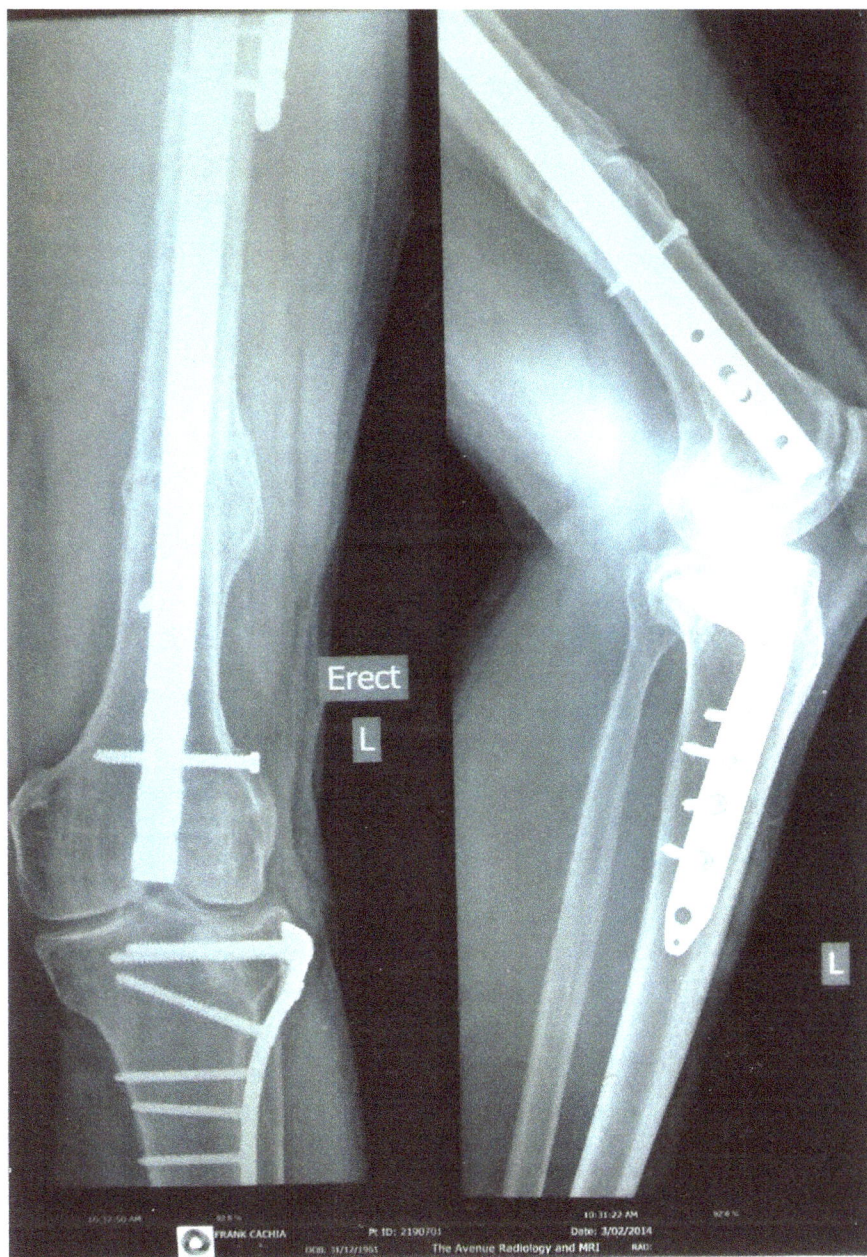

Yes, it was and is quite painful.

In between operations with practically no physical activity I became a couch potato. Although during this period I wrote 2 adult and 5 children's books about birds and successfully researched and completed both my parents Family Tree; the downside was that I passed time by raiding the pantry. Putting on weight was inevitable.

To make it worse, the side effect triggered by the multitude of pain killing tablets resulted in a partial loss of taste. This developed in the inability of not being able to actually feel that I had had enough food. The outcome, eat even more and the weight kept on piling up.

While dressing to attend lunch on Christmas 2013, I had to (once again) suck in my stomach to do up my pants and belt. This was becoming an everyday occurrence and I found myself looking away from the dressing mirror. I had to admit that I was putting on weight and I decided that I should start to diet in the New Year. Ha, I casually 'forgot' to start dieting, so much for a New Year resolution.

In February 2014, on the 14th to be precise while camping with friends, I was in agony as my back was killing me. Still I put on a brave face when my mate took a photo of me. I was shocked with what I saw. No excuses this time, I not only promised, but did start to diet when I arrived back home. The first thing I did was to buy a (weighing) set of scales. That was a waste of money; with the stomach blocking the view I couldn't see the digital readout. I shook my head in disgust.

Four months later at an outdoor function, it was pointed out in no uncertain terms that I'm fat. Whether I liked it or not, no matter what excuse I could muster to explain my state, the fact remained that not only my diet wasn't working but I have actually put on more weight.

So I optimistically changed to another diet. That would work I mused. It didn't.

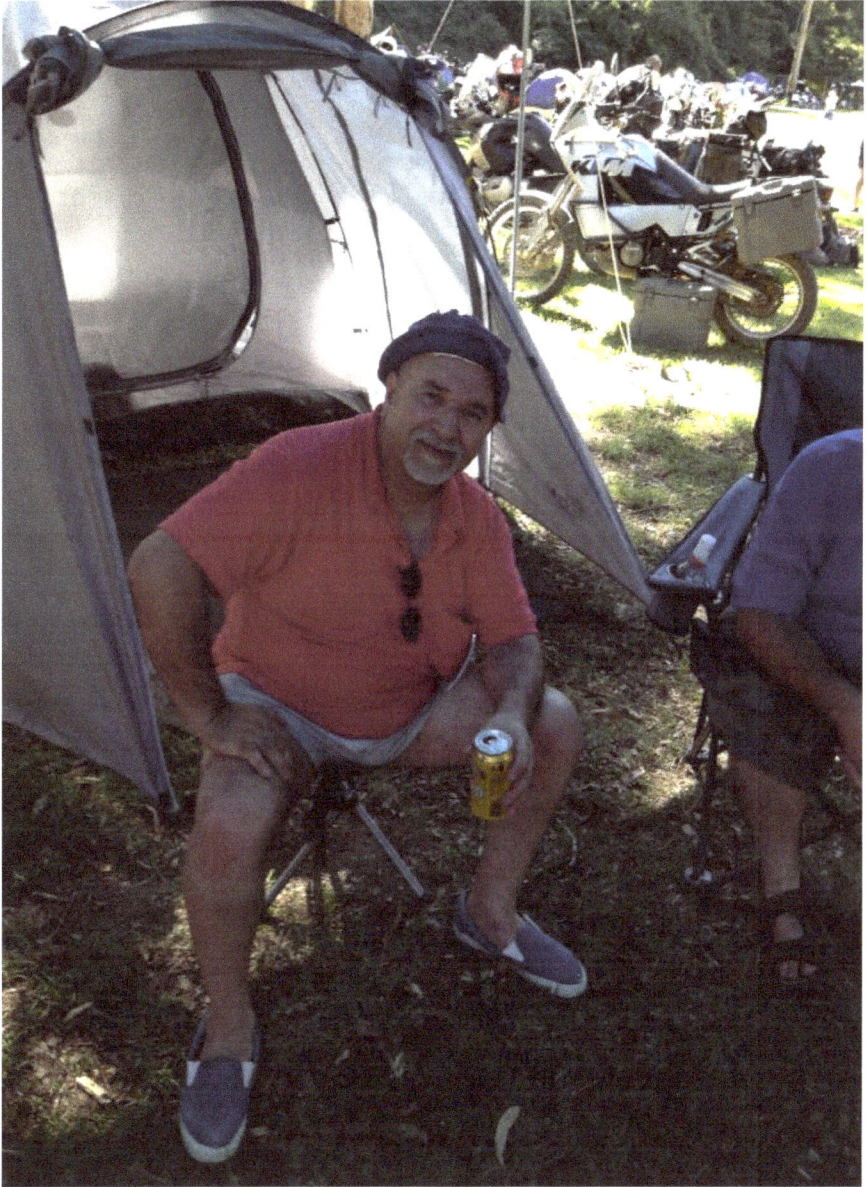

The Old Me

Complete Failure

After 3 months the result was more than just disappointing, it was downright demoralising. That winter, consuming a cold lunch and only another plain meal at night brought nothing but heartbreak. There was no weight reduction whatsoever. What did I have to do to lose weight? I tried another diet but with the same result-----no weight loss.

So I cut down even more, practically going into starvation mode. I did not know that going on a starvation diet results in the body trying to store more fat to be used in leaner times.

A month later I spoke to my doctor about my weight increase and asked him to point me to a professional. After taking a blood sample and checking my blood pressure he pointed me to a dietician. I was weighed and after paying close attention to her advice, I went home more optimistically, in the knowledge that I had been doing the wrong thing, in other words that I had no idea about dieting. So I started afresh.

Within a short time period without even trying, my weight started to drop. My confidence soared and I'm sure I was walking 6 inches off the ground.

What I had failed to accomplish in 8 months I succeeded in just on a month. Over time my body started to slim down and surprise, surprise, as time passed other noticeable changes started to emerge. These were benefits that I had never even thought of, let alone considered; I love it. I loved the changes taking place.

So what was this miracle diet? There isn't one; you see I wasn't on a diet at all. A diet is a reduction of calorific intake for a certain time period in an attempt at weight reduction. A change of eating habits however, is a lifetime change, a change in the quality and quantity of food, in other words, a different eating lifestyle.

Prepare to Succeed

Some people will tell you that it's poor urban planning or far too many fast takeaways that are to blame for putting on weight. Others will gladly point out that it is the computer's fault; meaning with so much technology around there's no time for exercise. What a lot of misguided advice.

Others mean well. The advice from friends and their helpful hints about dieting hasn't really helped. It's no one's fault, you see, the cause is that since school days we receive advice which is mostly incomplete or half true. The majority is either wrong, inaccurate or simply don't apply to you. Plus we choose to follow advice for our own reasons.

You know you need to lose weight; you have tried to do just that but have failed. This resulted in you going through a number of negative emotions. What's worse is that you most likely have increased in weight, but what's more distressing is losing faith in yourself. Naturally next time you attempt a "sure fire" diet, you subconsciously are preparing yourself to fail. So you start a vicious cycle.

Let me take you on a journey and share with you how effortlessly I lost weight----yes we are conditioned to believe that nothing is easy, but in this case it is, ridiculously easy.

Please keep in mind that I will on a number of occasions repeat certain statements. I do this to remind and emphasise.

The positive:

1. Believe in yourself. Accept this fact, only you can achieve your goal. Ask yourself this question----Do you believe you deserve less??

2. Look forward to the day a friend comments on the new you.

3. Nutrition information table. This is virtually the only guide you need to understand and follow. You'll be surprised how helpful this is.

4. Eating a wider range of food. You lose weight by eating more? This statement is a contradiction. But it's true, I learnt that to lose weight you'll find yourself looking for a wider range of products and eating more food.

The negative:

1. Doubt. Yep your first hurdle to overcome.

2. Temptation. Your eyes are bigger than your belly.

3. Excuses. Your weak spot, trying to justify your actions.

4. Losing weight is a stumbling block. No it isn't, even though you subconsciously think so.

5. Failure to lose weight isn't punishable but a clear sign to review where you might have 'tripped'.

6. Time, Sugar and Fat are your enemy.

Remember

1. Losing weight is just that, it applies to both male and female.

2. A complex issue of 2 different fat types and percentage fat ratios and their mobility is beyond the depth of this book.

3. Although it helps, you do not need to go jogging or take any other type of exercise to lose weight. Look at me; with a badly damaged leg I can hardly put much weight on it. My only exercise is riding an exercise bike to help keep the knee lubricated.

4. Increasing your metabolic rate by increased activity of any type increases your energy consumption and burns stored fat reserves.

5. Stress is a factor for gaining weight, because we turn to comfort foods when stressed. But if you continue using it as an excuse you'll never lose any weight. Similarly there's no tricks in losing weight but again always remember don't let any excuse justify your action.

6. Today living is usually done in the fast lane that still doesn't mean you should skip eating.

7. Don't let time rule you.

Time and Sugar – The Evil Twin

One Sunday I was sitting down at a roadside cafe with a couple. My lunch consisted of having two small sausage rolls and a glass of water. He had his usual egg, bacon, sausage and tomato roll and a cappuccino, while she stacked her plate to overflowing with a hamburger with the lot, a serving of French fries and washed down with a double chocolate milk shake. I was surprised to see the size of her plate. Wow, I said to myself, where she's going to fit all of that.

When I queried her choice of food, she pointed out that she needs to "fill up" as she plan to start a sure fire diet the following day. She then proceeded to explain that she's starting a diet that will cause her to lose 6kg in 6 weeks. Upon further questioning, she explained that she'll eat a variety of vegetables during the week and as much meat as she likes during the weekend. She said it's guaranteed to lose the weight.

I had no doubt that yes she'll lose weight initially, but in time will not only regain it and most likely even more. I wanted to ask her "What happens after the sixth and seventh week? What plans if any are implemented to tackle the following weeks? What happens in 2, 3 or 4 months? Instead I refrained from asking. Clearly her mind was made up and no discussion will change it.

This was a diet that a friend had passed onto her and blindly followed. Off course when the diet didn't work she started to feel a range of negative emotions and most likely blamed the diet or her friend. But the worst mistake is the most common that many people fall victim to by placing a Time Limit.

Why place a time limit, it's not a race? Nowhere does it say that when you lose weight you need a specific period of time. There are so many diets that specify a time period. When you lose weight correctly, it should be forever not just for a period of time.

You see with diets, any type of diet will work, while you follow it, you'll lose weight. But diets, any diet will eventually fail. Why is it so? Because when you stop, you resume your past eating habits.

Well simply put, if they did successfully work there wouldn't be so many around. The main reasons they fail is either because of time constraint or because they restrict certain foods that has been recognised by the tongue for decades. The body will demand and unless you have the will power of a statue will send a message to the brain to desire, want, and demand said items. The brain will argue first logically then emotionally and eventually uses any excuse to justify the action. The diet will fail and guilt will surface.

Sugar

Calories, Carbohydrates and Sugar.

Looking up the definition it says:

> Calories are units of energy. Various definitions exist but fall into two broad categories. The small calorie or gram calorie is the approximate amount of energy needed to raise the temperature of one gram of water by one degree Celsius at a pressure of one atmosphere.

Do you have an idea what this means?? Do you really care?

It also says:

That an average woman needs to eat about 2000 calories per day and an average man needs an extra 500 calories. What's average? Define average? What happens if you go over the allotted number? The last thing I wanted to do before sitting down to enjoy eating is to do some arithmetic. I could just imagine looking at a mouthful of food and then spend time add this to this, then subtract this amount, before dividing by such and such.

Forget it, what a cruel way to spoil ones appetite.

This is as bad as trying to workout carbohydrates. Carbohydrates are found in a wide variety of foods. The important sources are cereals, potatoes, fruits, table sugar = sucrose = cane sugar, bread, milk, etc.

Nice to know but all these words achieve is a headache.

So for the moment disregard all the advice thrown at you and concentrate on *reducing* the REFINED AND PROCESSED SUGAR content, after all that's an enemy of the worse kind, if not the worse enemy you have facing you when trying to lose weight.

To any observer it looked like I did absolutely nothing different in the first month of my new life. In actual fact I did something that I should have done decades if not a lifetime before. I used to take 2 ½ heaped teaspoons of sugar in my coffee and tea. I began very minutely and I do mean very minutely, reducing the amount using a measuring spoon. It was so little that I didn't even notice it. However, there was a major drop by the end of the month.

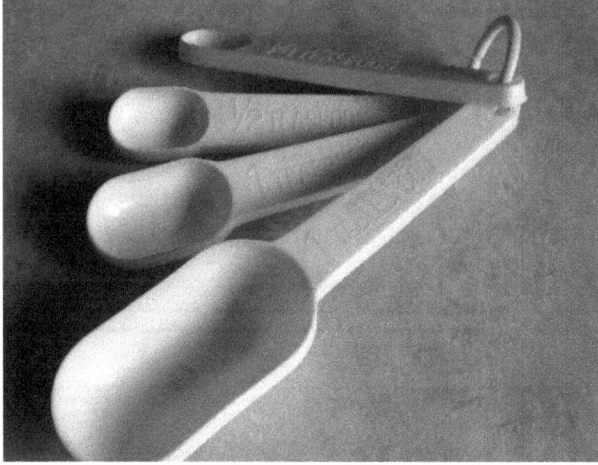

Nothing else had changed; I'm still eating the same. Still drinking coffee and tea but I'm starting to educate my taste buds. And because I'm doing it painfully slow the body doesn't miss the drop in quantity. Just quickly moving ahead I'm now using just a ¼ of a teaspoon having successfully dropped a total of 2 ¼ teaspoons per cup. And occasionally, when I have absentmindedly forgotten to actually use any sugar I just went right ahead and drank my drink without any sugar at all.

This is perhaps the most difficult thing to give up but at a dead slow pace it's quite easy. Remember you're not in a race.

Sugar should be classified as a drug. Why? Because it is so addictive, its sweetness and ease of availability wants us to want more.

As children we were given sugar in the form of sweets as a reward or a bribe. In days gone by even the dentist, of all people, gave us a lolly after a visit. And let's not forget birthday cakes with all that icing. It is also comforting. Ha, no wonder we're hooked on it! We love it, desire and want it. We never stood a chance.

Our body wants it as it quickly converts it to energy. The problem is that unless it is used up, the body will store it for later use and that is the main problem; too much of it causes weight increase. Therefore, logic dictates that by reducing our sugar intake this should lead to our weight reducing.

As mentioned, the body stores sugar. However it cannot be stored as sugar. Our bodies convert sugar into a safe product known as fat that can easily be converted back to sugar when needed. If we over indulge on it no amount of exercise will help. Refined sugar is your worse enemy.

There's another reason we should reduce our added sugar intake. All surplus energy including that found in sugar in all its forms will be converted to fat. Surplus energy which the body converts to fat that will accumulate around vital organs and in time cause those affected to hinder their functions.

By the way, whether it is processed or refined or raw or even natural, sugar is sugar. This includes alcoholic liquor as the alcohol content is derived from sugar fermenting. The energy remains and once in the body must be processed to a safe product = Fat. So for overall well-being start reducing or I should say start to shy away from such a drug.

And finally although reducing sugar will see a drop in weight don't expect to see the loss straight away.

Just as I started to educate the palate about sugar other habits followed. For example I'll still eat a slice of cake when offered but then I'll abstain from a coffee for the day. Don't expect to do just this suddenly, but you'll find that you'll do this in the future. So once again I stress the point, you're not 'short changing' yourself, just backing away thus giving your body time to not only adjust but give it a longer period of time in between such sugary intakes.

Reminder, although there was hardly any drop in weight, over a full month that drops is noticeable. Once you weigh yourself, I'll guarantee that you too will walk 6 inches off the ground carrying a smile on your face and a song in your heart.

The most significant change of note is a change of attitude. As hard as it is to believe, you'll actually start to 'Police' yourself. You'll start to become aware of your eating habits and question what you're eating.

Multiple Meals

On an average day, I eat 4 - 5 meals

Breakfast

We can survive on just plain food, but it becomes quite bland after a while. Thanks to a wide range of taste buds, we add all sorts of other foods and flavourings to help improve the taste making the experience of eating not only nourishing but help the medication 'go down'.

The first meal of the day, the meal that they say is the most important meal of the day; we have a wide selection to choose from. Unfortunately, breakfast time is running around, both for you and perhaps your family is in a state of pandemonium; you're on automatic pilot. You end up eating the same food day in day out.

Stop because now, before you take your first bite, it's time to pause, look, and plan and change your eating habits. It's time to enter the world of Nutritional Information Tables. Using this as a guide you'll not only start to lose weight but find yourself as previously stated eating a wider range of food. Yes you'll start to lose weight by eating more?

Nutritional Information is nothing more than the information displayed on a wide variety of supermarket products. Use the information displayed, it will tell you what to safely have, what to briefly avoid and what to stay away from. Remember, in this weight loss, there's not one product that we should completely abstain from.

We do not need processed sugar in our diet. There are many natural sugars in many foods that we consume.

For the moment forget all you see except for the "Sugars" listed below the Carbohydrate. The last column has a figure of less than 1g this is definitely one product that I'll consume.

SERVINGS PER PACKAGE – 40 SERVING SIZE – 250mL	WHEN MADE UP AS DIRECTED (1 PART CORDIAL TO 4 PARTS WATER)		
AVERAGE PER SERVING:	250mL	%DI*	100mL
ENERGY	32kJ	0.4%	13kJ
PROTEIN	0g	0%	0g
FAT – TOTAL	0g	0%	0g
– SATURATED	0g	0%	0g
CARBOHYDRATE	1.2g	0.4%	LESS THAN 1g
– SUGARS	1.1g	1%	LESS THAN 1g
DIETARY FIBRE	0.2g	0.1%	0.1g
SODIUM	25mg	1%	10mg
VITAMIN C	5mg	13%(†RDI)	2mg

*PERCENTAGE DAILY INTAKES ARE BASED ON AN AVERAGE ADULT

A Very Friendly Nutritional Information Table

You can select any figure you like as a guide. I aim for less than 15g per 100g. Why? Because it is quite a low sugar content, yet not that low to make it so restrictive to anything else. Have a look at the following labels and you can see the difference of sugar content in everyday products.

SERVINGS PER PACKAGE: 11   SERVING SIZE: 23.2 g (4 BISCUITS)

	AVG. QUANTITY PER SERVING	% DAILY INTAKE* (PER SERVING)	AVG. QUANTITY PER 100 g
ENERGY	397 kJ	4.6%	1,710 kJ
PROTEIN	2.8 g	5.7%	12.2 g
FAT, TOTAL	2.2 g	3.1%	9.4 g
-SATURATED	0.3 g	1.1%	1.1 g
-TRANS	0.0 g		0.1 g
-POLYUNSATURATED	0.9 g		3.8 g
-MONOUNSATURATED	1.0 g		4.3 g
CHOLESTEROL	0 mg		0 mg
CARBOHYDRATE	14.5 g	4.7%	62.3 g
-SUGARS	0.4 g	0.5%	1.8 g
DIETARY FIBRE	2.8 g	9.3%	12.0 g
SODIUM	105 mg	4.6%	452 mg
NIACIN VIT(B3)	1.7 mg (17%)†		7.4 mg

A packet of Vita Weet

NUTRITION INFORMATION:
Servings per package: Approx. 12   Serving size: 20g

	Avg. Quantity Per serving	% Daily Intake* Per serving	Avg. Quantity Per 100g
Energy	175kJ (42Cal)	2%	875kJ (209Cal)
Protein	0.1g	0.2%	0.3g
Fat, total	LESS THAN 0.1g	0%	0.2g
- saturated	LESS THAN 0.1g	0%	0.1g
Carbohydrate	10.0g	3%	50.0g
- sugars	9.5g	11%	47.5g
Dietary Fibre, total	0.3g	1%	1.5g
Sodium	2mg	0%	8mg

* Percentage Daily Intakes are based on an average adult diet of 8700kJ. Your daily intakes may be

Strawberry Fruit Spread at 47.5g

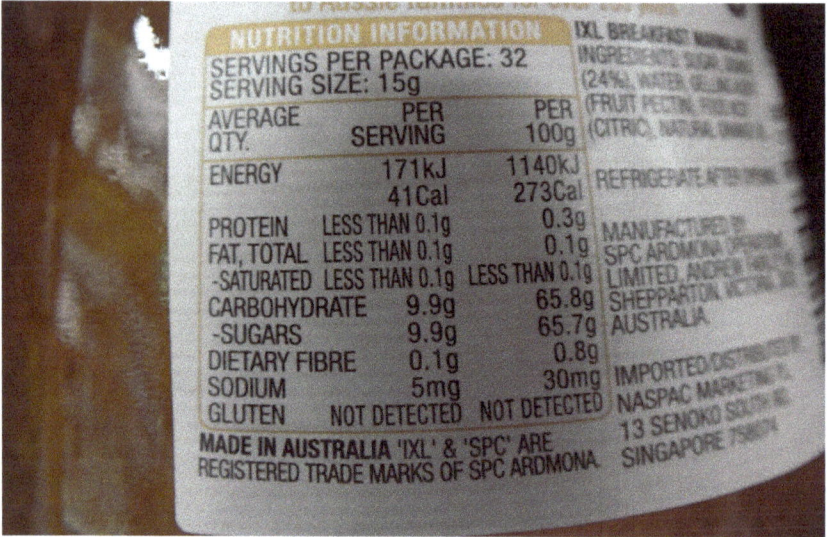

Apricot Jam at 65g that's a bit much

NUTRITION INFORMATION			
SERVINGS PER PACKAGE: 32			
SERVING SIZE: 15g			
AVERAGE QTY.	PER SERVING	PER 100g	
ENERGY	171kJ	1140kJ	
	41Cal	273Cal	
PROTEIN	LESS THAN 0.1g	0.3g	
FAT, TOTAL	LESS THAN 0.1g	0.1g	
-SATURATED	LESS THAN 0.1g	LESS THAN 0.1g	
CARBOHYDRATE	9.9g	65.8g	
-SUGARS	9.9g	65.7g	
DIETARY FIBRE	0.1g	0.8g	
SODIUM	5mg	30mg	
GLUTEN	NOT DETECTED	NOT DETECTED	

MADE IN AUSTRALIA 'IXL' & 'SPC' ARE REGISTERED TRADE MARKS OF SPC ARDMONA.

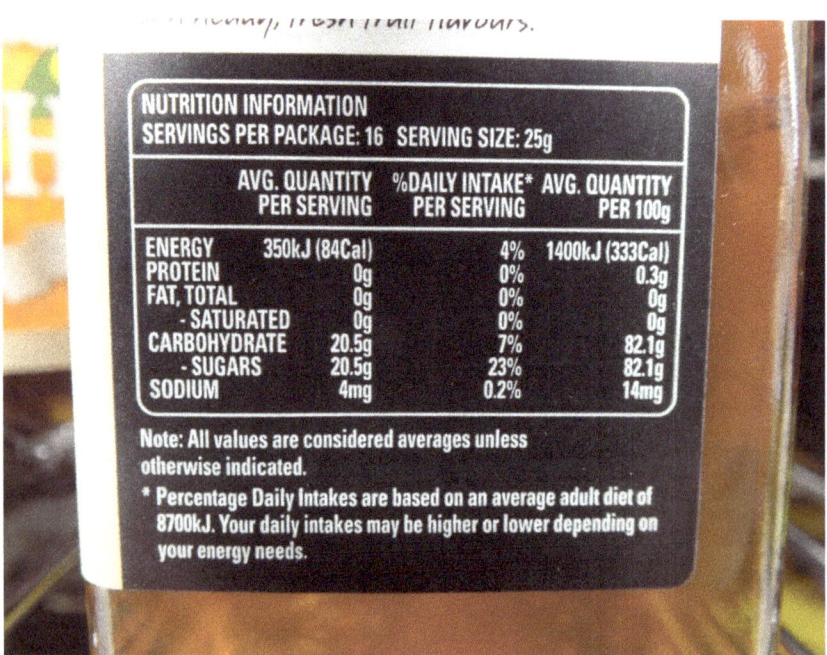

At 82g that's definitely way too high

NUTRITION INFORMATION			
SERVINGS PER PACKAGE: 16 SERVING SIZE: 25g			
	AVG. QUANTITY PER SERVING	%DAILY INTAKE* PER SERVING	AVG. QUANTITY PER 100g
ENERGY	350kJ (84Cal)	4%	1400kJ (333Cal)
PROTEIN	0g	0%	0.3g
FAT, TOTAL	0g	0%	0g
- SATURATED	0g	0%	0g
CARBOHYDRATE	20.5g	7%	82.1g
- SUGARS	20.5g	23%	82.1g
SODIUM	4mg	0.2%	14mg

Note: All values are considered averages unless otherwise indicated.

* Percentage Daily Intakes are based on an average adult diet of 8700kJ. Your daily intakes may be higher or lower depending on your energy needs.

Clearly of all the toppings, I'd select the one with the lowest sugar content, the Strawberry Fruit Spread at 47.5g. As it is still way above my 15g limit than I'll use it only sparingly AND for only 2 maybe 3 days per week. On alternate mornings, I altogether change and have a completely different type of breakfast. You see I'm modifying my eating habits without short changing myself. This way I'm still eating, still enjoying the topping but am regulating the frequency. I'm giving the body time to burn off the energy in the sugar and because it is quite sparingly consumed, not giving the body much sugar/energy to store.

This particular morning apart from a cup of tea, I ate an English muffin with vegemite and strawberry fruit spread. Have a look and see how little I use.

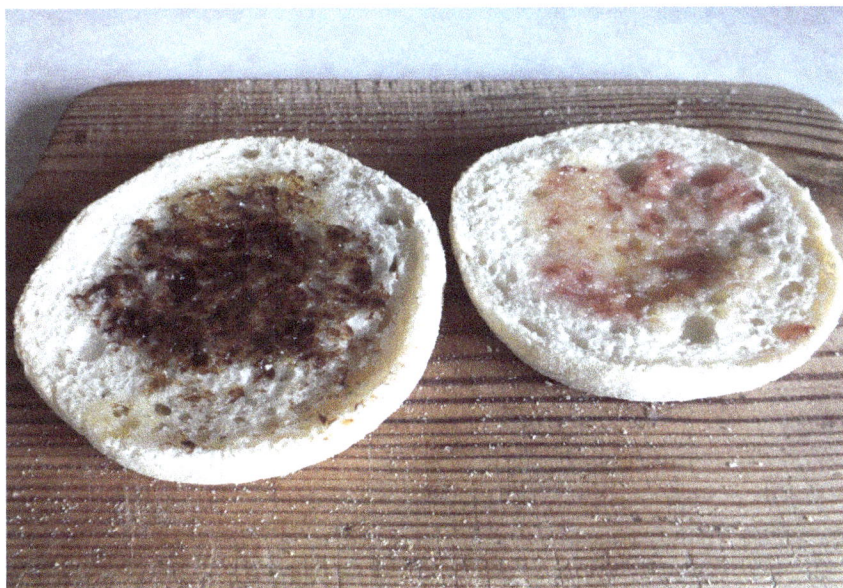

"Breakfast of Champions?"

Now the first thing you'll think is "I can't survive on just that, I'll still be hungry" And you're right; don't try this on your first day, it simply isn't enough, but one day it will. So for the moment eat four muffins and believe me, one day without even trying your stomach will say, nah, four is becoming too much, I'll just settle for three, then a little later, two. And you can't but help policing yourself. You're on a roll.

I wash this muffin down with the delicious cup of tea. Remember I was putting 2 ½ heaps of teaspoons of sugar and I said I slowly dropped down to just ¼, well here it is.

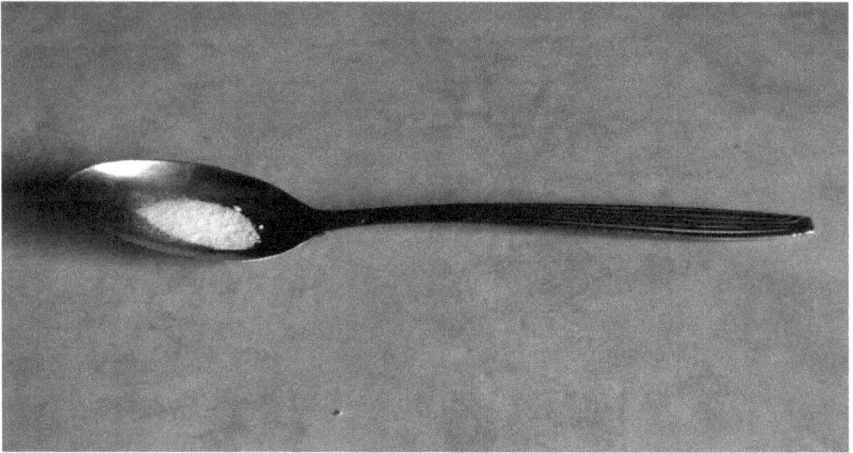

Eventually this is enough sugar

You may remember how I said you'll start to question what you're eating. Have a look at the English muffin and see if you can spot what's missing. It's quite obvious, hardly any butter and none on the vegemite one. I stopped using this product. I weened myself of it. Why? Well I'm using the muffin to ease my appetite and the vegemite and strawberry fruit spread for taste, something that is deliciously pleasing to me and my palate.

So why do I need butter or worse, margarine? Once you have spread the jam or any similar other produce, as long as no one is watching, you'll mostly likely lick the utensil. Why, because of the delicious taste. But you wouldn't do that to a smear of margarine, because let's face it, unless it is salted, it's a bland taste. So if we accept that yes it is a bland taste, why use it?

The same applies if you, say make a sandwich with ham, cheese, tomato and lettuce. You have four strong tastes to enjoy and those tastes are strong enough to mask the taste of margarine, so why spread it, why use it?

Incidentally while I'm on the same subject, it's time to point out NOT to rely too heavily on advertising slogans. The best example I can show you is where the manufacturer claims that the product is 99% fat free. That might be quite true, but what's the size of volume of the other 1%?

I mentioned salt; it's worth noting that salt makes your body hold on to water. If you eat too much salt, the extra salt stored in your body forces your body to retain fluids thus raises your blood pressure. So, the more salt you eat, the higher your blood pressure. Apart from a medical point of view, this definitely doesn't help when you're trying to lose weight.

STRAWBERRY NUTRITION INFORMATION			
SERVINGS PER TUB: 1		SERVING SIZE: 175g	
	AVE. QTY. PER SERVE	%DI* AVE. QTY. PER SERVE	PER 100g
ENERGY	275kJ (66 Cal)	3%	157kJ (38Cal)
PROTEIN, TOTAL	7.5g	15%	4.3g
- GLUTEN	0mg		0mg
FAT, TOTAL	0.2g	0%	0.1g
- SATURATED	0.2g	1%	0.1g
CARBOHYDRATE	8.4g	3%	4.8g
- SUGARS	7.7g	9%	4.4g
- ADDED SUGARS	0g		0g
DIETARY FIBRE	2.6g	9%	1.5g
SODIUM	96mg	4%	55mg
CALCIUM	254mg	32% RDI*	145mg

STRAWBERRY INGREDIENTS:
SKIM MILK MILK

Friendly Yogurt

To avoid boredom with a limited diet, I altogether change and have a completely different type of breakfast. Yes, I treat my palate to a complete change. I'm still eating, I haven't backed off and gone on a hunger or starvation mode, I'd just change my breakfast menu.

With my cup of tea I'll have a banana and a tub of yoghurt. Since yoghurt only has a low 4.4g of sugar you can lash out and have more tubs. In time you'll gradually reduce down to just one.

Alternate the meals and change again to say a refreshing orange or a mango and different flavoured yoghurt. Go for a hard-boiled egg and a slice of toast and an apricot. Now if you say "oh what a mix up", where does it say that you have to regiment your breakfast? The aim here is that you're not feeling hungry and you are not losing interest in monotonous repeat meals as other diets eventually tend to do so; you're still eating and better yet, still enjoying food.

Toast is quite nice with numerous choices of toppings. Try a fruit loaf with sunflower seeds from the local bakery. Two slices are enough, quite filling and yummy to boot.

Incidentally it's time to point out that you should also place a restriction on the amount of fruit as a daily consumption. Fruit, irrespective how good it is still has sugar in it. Yes it is natural sugar but still sugar, and sugar in all form is still sugar. I have limited myself to no more than 3 pieces of fruit a day. It must be right, it works.

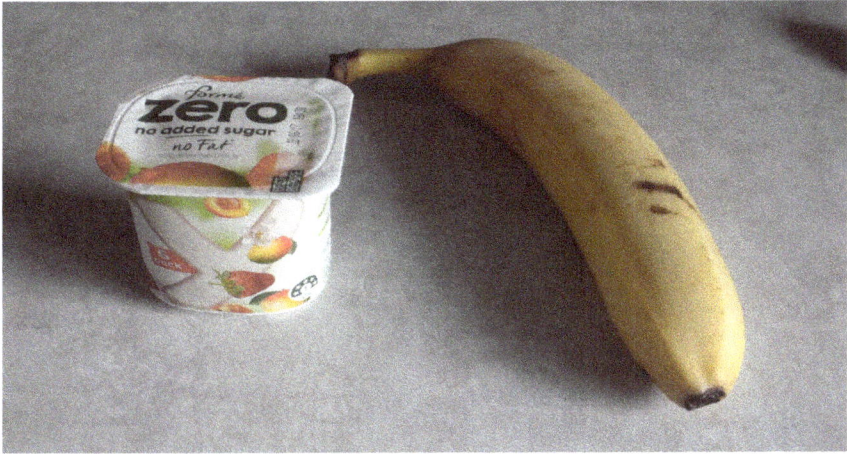

Quite Satisfactory

Do not fool yourself that by juggling food around it will help your weight loss.

Two perfectly good examples:

At a wayside stop I observed a person eat six sugar covered jam donuts. Knowing full well that he has consumed quite a lot of sugar he ordered a diet soft drink. No, that doesn't balance the sugar contents.

One person without fail daily consumes a full English breakfast. His plate has 2 eggs, 2 strips of fried bacon, 2 fried sausages, 2 Fried tomatoes, 2 fried potatoes, and 3 slices of fried bread in fat juices, some mushrooms and baked beans. A glass of orange juice and a cup of tea followed. When I pointed out to him that that this is way too much and worse it's all fried, he commented that it is his national breakfast. When I said that he should change his eating habit he agreed to remove the mushrooms and toast his 3 slices of bread. I laughed; I said that all he's doing is negotiating over food. I pointed out that if he's serious in losing weight arguing over traditional meals isn't an issue. This isn't up for a bartering chat, it's not a short term weight loss; it's a change in eating lifestyle.

So do not stick with a routine, expand your palate, be adventurous and try out new tastes. All you have to lose is weight.

Now that breakfast is over, usually tradition dictates a lunch and finally a dinner. Well for me that wasn't enough. If you want to lose weight you'll have to eat more frequent smaller meals. It's true, eating more will help you lose weight. Remember when I said "consuming a cold lunch and only another meal at night" well I was so wrong----how so?

In a nutshell, the stomach role is to digest and process food. As long as it's working you can't get hunger pains. If, like I was doing, eating only two meals a day then the stomach was empty for quite a considerable amount of time. Eventually you'll get hunger signals and feel the need to have a 'hearty' meal. Therefore by increasing food intake, at a reduced size, thus reducing the period between meals the stomach is less likely to become hungry thus impeding hunger pains.

I eat up to 5 small meals a day. I'm never hungry, just on the rare occasion a bit peckish.

When able to, I'll have breakfast, lunch, afternoon tea, dinner and supper. On average, I eat every four hours. Remember I said when able to. If I do miss one I'll try to eat something an hour later. If not than I will eat when due but making sure than I do not increase the amount of food intake to 'compensate'. I don't have to have a big meal because four hours later I'll be eating again.

A friend who at times does interstate runs always helped himself to a humongous breakfast in the belief that it will sustain him for hour upon hour. All he succeeded in doing was stretch his stomach resulting in his stomach wanting a bigger meal to feel that it has been given the same quantity.

Remember when we were young and our parents told us off for having a bite to eat saying "you'll spoil your dinner" Well that is precisely what we should be doing. By eating more regularly each portion is less because the stomach doesn't need a lot, it isn't empty.

Lunch

You start having lunch just like you always have. But by changing to a new eating lifestyle, just like a change in breakfast, lunch changes too. Before I started dieting, I would eat five slices of white bread covered in butter, and a slice of ham, cheese, tomato, lettuce, pickle and topped up with a dash of mayonnaise. A bubbly soft drink, a small block of chocolate and a banana followed. When I started my first diet, I immediately stopped and ate a banana and an apple. What was an enjoyable meal turned to nothing more than a one minute event. Within a few weeks I stopped looking forward to it. Lunch became nothing more than a bland meal, if you can even call it that. To make it worse within an hour I felt peckish and had only about eight hours before my next (self-imposed) meal. Dinner was not a meal to enjoy rather than an exercise in stuffing myself because by then I was quite ravenous.

Now with only a few hours between meals, I plan my small, light meal, looking forward to see what culinary delights are in store. Mmmmm, what shall I have, there's just so much tasty food available. And they all have little or hardly any sugar.

Instead of white or any other bread for that matter, I now have 2 slices of what's called Corn Thins and place a slice of Silverside, with the fat trimmed away, on top of a slice of low fat cheese.

Accompanying this delicious meal, 2 Vita-Weet biscuits each are adorned with a slice of Strasbourg meat. An apple makes up the rest of this banquet. It is more than enough. There's hardly any sugar, it is filling, most satisfying and quite delicious.

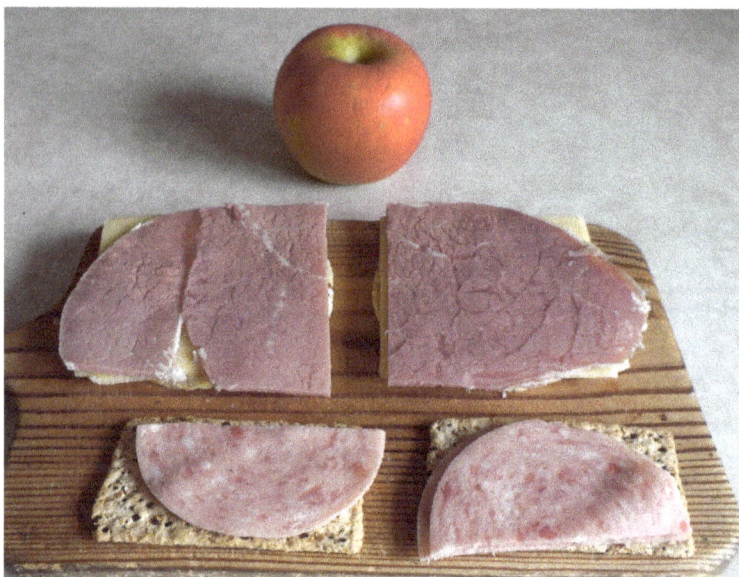

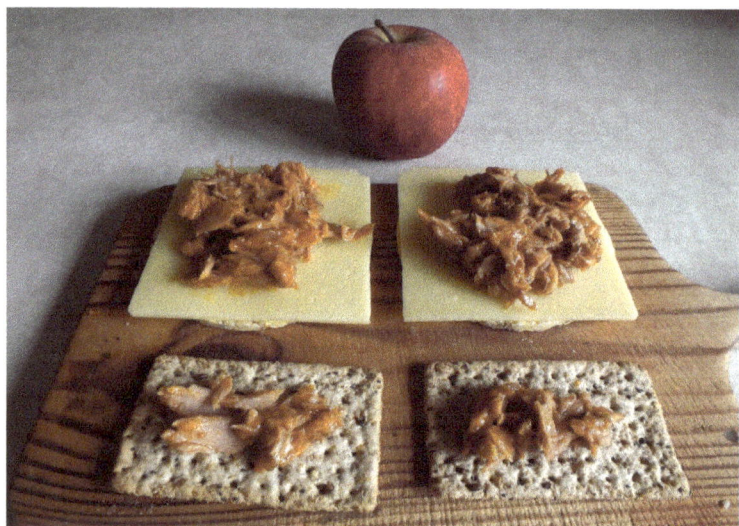

Variations of the Same Theme

Again, notice the lack of butter or margarine.

To give my taste buds another treat, using the same base, a couple of Ryvita biscuits can be substituted for the Vita-Weet. But if I'm really going to lash out and live it up, still using the same base add a slice of tomatoes or better yet, how about a small can of salmon or tuna atop those slices of cheese? Another apple wouldn't hurt, neither would an orange.

So once again you're enjoying a meal without putting on any weight. Again as you read this you think it's not enough but remember as you lose weight you will not eat as much. In my case this is enough. I'm now at a point that if I'm out to lunch, a single solitary sausage roll plus a cappuccino is more than ample.

Afternoon tea

By now another few hours have passed since lunch so give yourself a break and enjoy a very light snack together with a nice cup of tea or coffee. It doesn't have to be much; all you're doing is keeping your stomach active thus keeping hunger signals at bay.

Once again, I turn to a corn thin and a Vita Weet with a touch of vegemite and corn relish or fruit chutney. As the toppings contain sugar apply sparingly and it's quite tasty. I change the bases and toppings frequently giving my taste buds a treat.

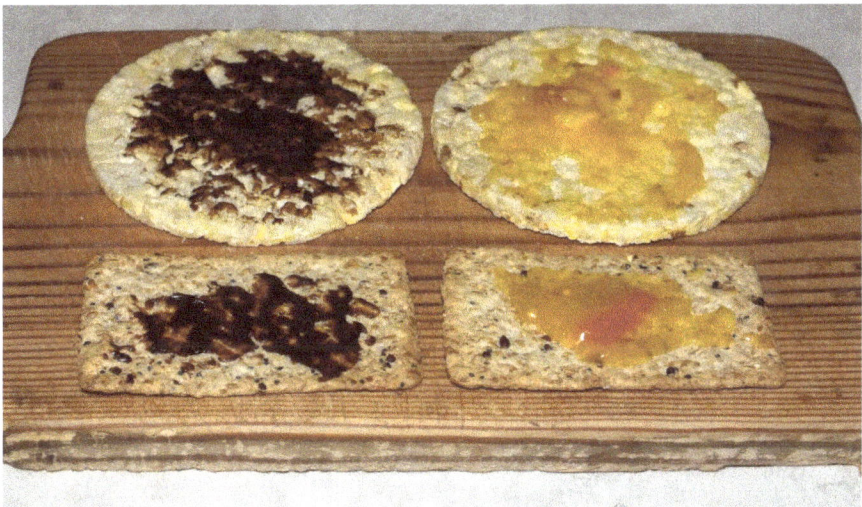

Simple and Enjoyable

A walk down a supermarket isle will reveal all sorts of delicious spreads. All you have to do is keep an eye on the sugar content.

Dinner

So far, all foods consumed today have been relatively light both in sugar, fat and quantity. There's no reason why dinner or tomorrows food intake should be any difference. In my case I mix and match all sorts of food varieties ranging from meat, pasta, rice and vegetables. On occasion, I sprinkle a sauce or salt and pepper. I'm definitely not short changing myself.

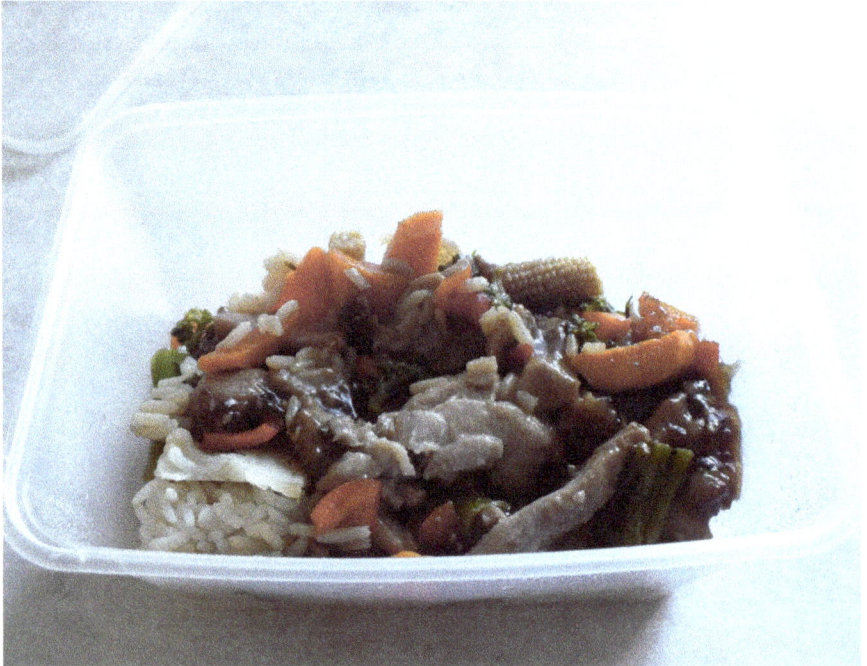

Dinner - Chicken, Vegetables and Rice

For a time, to ensure that I did not cook too much, thus preventing me from overeating, I used to prepare the meal in a standard size food plastic container. This resulted in having everything measured. To help yourself along, remember the following often overheard statements:

1. "Clean up your plate"

2. "Waste not, want not".

By measuring, meaning controlling your intake, the above statements wouldn't apply.

I started with a full container, now with the weight loss; a full container is way too much.

Now this meal can easily be washed down with a coffee, a wine or even a spirit. Yes if you do want any of these drinks, by all means do have some, and enjoy them. A change of lifestyle doesn't mean abstaining; what you should do since sugar can be found in any of these drinks is to ease off the amount or the frequency.

Dinner is now over, the washed dishes are put away and it's time to relax watching TV. This, mostly, is the time to nibble on sweets or chocolate. And this unfortunately is also the time were too much sugar and fat is consumed. All the good you have done during the day is wasted.

What's even worse is if friends drop by and you'll bring out a selection of cheeses and crackers. What's even worse still is the range of other nibbles such as chips and dips.

If you want to lay out a spread do so, but abstain from indulging to excess yourself. Let others help themselves, be happy in the knowledge that you're on a mission. So how do you not feel left out? Join in by consuming some grapes. Not many, no more than say 10 - 15. You're still 'in with the crowd' but your sugar intake is very minimal. And keep in mind that, that is the third and last fruit for the day.

Now let's imagine that no friends dropped in, and all you have touched were a handful of grapes. Time has passed and now you're ready for bed. You can now safely turn in, smiling in the knowledge that you have 'won'. You haven't felt hungry, having eaten four times of four meals. You have drastically reduced the sugar intake and you are looking forward, and this is extremely important, to a new breakfast in a few hours. By now you are dictating eating terms, not your stomach.

Alas you are starting to feel peckish. Now is the time to say NO – Enough: after all you haven't exercised any will power throughout the day. This is all very well but what happens if there's a lack of will power? Then go to the fridge and have some more fruit.

I use to have a can of pineapple? It is quite refreshing, quite filling and the sugar content is in the 'safe zone'. To make certain that the sugar remains in the safe zone have the small 4 slice rather than the big 9 slice can. A banana or an apple will do as good a job.

Now you'll say "oh no that's the fourth piece of fruit, I've gone over the limit". First things first, do not feel guilty. A slip is just that, a slip, a minor detail. Next time it happens, cut up a banana in half and eat that. By eating such a tiny amount, it's definitely not hurting you, it's satisfying the taste buds and it helps ease the guilt. It works, it really works.

This feeling peckish just before you turn in will not happen every day. As you naturally lose weight, as I said, your success will cause you to police yourself by reducing the amount consumed. Even the hunger pains reduce in severity.

Temptation

The day is now over so have a good night sleep. Tomorrow your new outlook on food will be another adventure.

It's easy to say, all is well, and have a good night sleep. The worse part of losing weight is The Temptation. The mind, the mouth and the stomach will play numerous tricks to satisfying the taste buds. So the best thing to do is take the time to end temptation. How you may ask? It's so easy, by the only way possible. To give up temptation, give in to it.

The best way to fight temptation is to reward, by tempting yourself. Yep, you heard right, use temptation as a reward. By placing temptation in front of you, you are now able to control it rather than letting it control you.

Off course certain foods are so delicious to the palate that you do not want to give it up. Regrettably this is where failure to lose weight occurs. The person who has, say a weakness for a certain product tries to stop, does partially succeed, but eventually weakens and unable to resist, eats the desired food. Believing failure, gives up, ends up feeling so remorseful that will completely stop dieting. That starts a downhill spiral.

So what do you do? Easy, have some. Yes, it is that simple have some, after all why should you short-change yourself? But, yes, there's always a 'But'.

Let's use a product which has very high sugar content as an example. This is a product that you simply love to have say, on your toast. There are a number of steps to continue eating it whilst still losing weight.

Reduce the amount. Instead of placing a thick layer, reduce the volume. After all the tongue doesn't know any better. Having a thick layer isn't going to increase the taste, that still remains the same.

Time; a time frame is nothing more that instead of having it every day, slowly over a period of say a month have it every second day, than slow down to every fourth day and so on. It isn't hard because you are slowly educating the taste buds to do without. Remember that's how I dropped my sugar content in coffee and tea. At the same time, substitute the product with another, a new taste, making sure it has lower sugar content.

Most likely by the end of the month you'll do without this favourite product. So in time look forward to have some, have it as a reward. Yes reward yourself for 'being good' by having the most desirable thing you love to have. You're still losing weight, you're still enjoying the taste, you're still eating it, but now you dictate the time and place and size of portion, not the other way round.

In effect you're fighting fire with fire. Reward yourself.

I reward myself every day. Twice a week I have a cup of soup with my dinner. On Wednesday, I buy takeaway, my favourite is Chinese takeaway to be precise. Since prawn crackers are fried, than I get some every second or third week. A handful of grapes are also enjoyed. Come Sunday it's a small bowl of yummy chocolate ice cream.

There was a time when after dinner sitting in front of the computer, I had a coffee, a big block of chocolate and a glass of Port. Now I have the same although quite a small portion compared to what I used to have, and I have them in a longer interval. I don't miss them at all. As a matter of fact, I was given a box of 6 chocolates as a Christmas gift. Since they were individually wrapped, I had one with dinner on the first day of every month. Why such a long period between bites? Easy, I'm having a small serve of chocolate ice cream once a week.

And finally the unexpected side benefits of weight loss.

At the very beginning of this book, I stated that I successfully reached and passed my weight limit. At the time I weighed 97kg. When asked how much weight I wanted to lose, I had no idea, I had never even thought of reaching any figure, I just wanted to lose weight. It was suggested that I should aim to 'turn' the numbers around. I said OK so I aimed to reach 79kg. That's a drop of 18kg. There was never a talk about a time limit.

As I said, I did it so easily, so effortlessly that at the last weigh-in, I easily passed my limit and have now lost a total of 26.1kgs. That's close to a quarter of my body weight. Whereas at Christmas 2013, I had to suck in my stomach to do up the pants and belt, now I have to push my stomach out to hold my pants from falling, so I can do up the belt. This was a personal victory.

Now when I'm at a function and I am faced with a choice of a slice of strawberry Pavlova, Chocolate cake, Black Forest cake or a fruit salad, I select the fruit salad. Not for fear of putting on weight, but because a fruit salad offers a multitude of tastes. Another reason, is because I've now conditioned myself to go to a better, more taster choice. Without really trying to dictate terms, temptation has become a thing of the past.

At the same time, I could have easily gone the other way and help myself to any of the cakes knowing full well that I will not gain any weight for the simple reason that I have proved beyond a shadow of doubt that I can easily lose the weight without even trying.

A Pleasant Surprise

A number of benefits appeared as I slowly shed weight.

One day my physiotherapist pointed out that I have stopped complaining of back aches. Although at times the lower back does act up, gone are the days of crippling pain. More interestingly, he pointed out that I have gained an exceptional amount of spinal flexibility.

My Physio and his wife spent a lot of time coaching me on my early dietary understanding, before I started with the Dietitian.

When attending my dentist for the dental inspection, he hasn't found any teeth that require any fillings. More so he pointed out that my gums are quite healthy.

My doctor is very happy with me. Blood tests show that my cholesterol has dropped quite significantly by around 45% to be exact. But to him the highlight has been my blood pressure. The day before I started my weight loss, he took my blood pressure. It was 159/127. The last time he took a reading it was 118/68. He cried out, 'excellent', smiled and said that I have the blood pressure of a child. Not bad for a 65 year old man!!

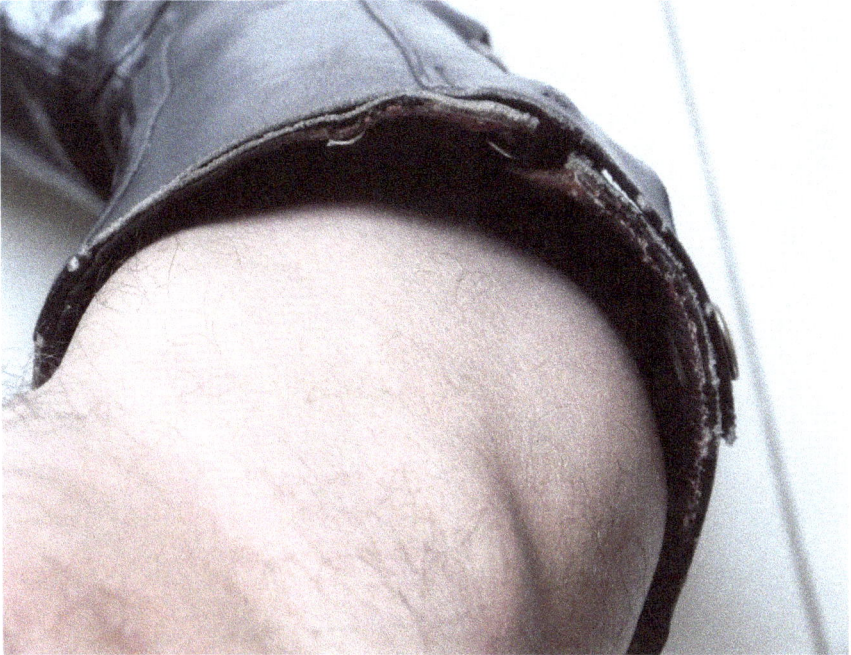

Other parts of the body such as the legs Lose Weight as well.

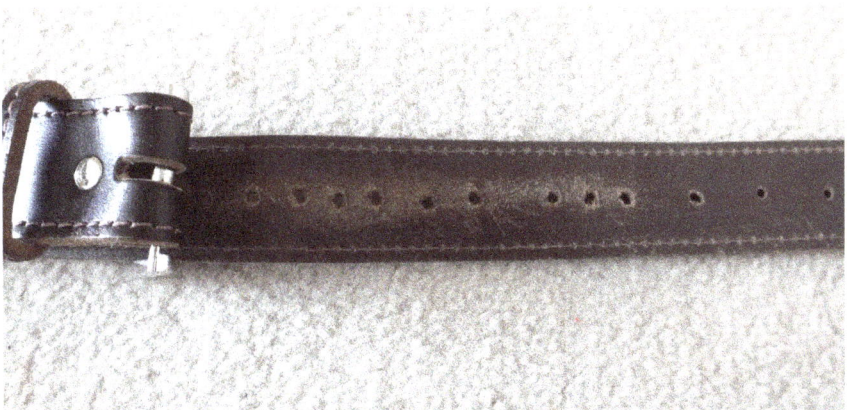

As weight started to drop the belt required more holes.

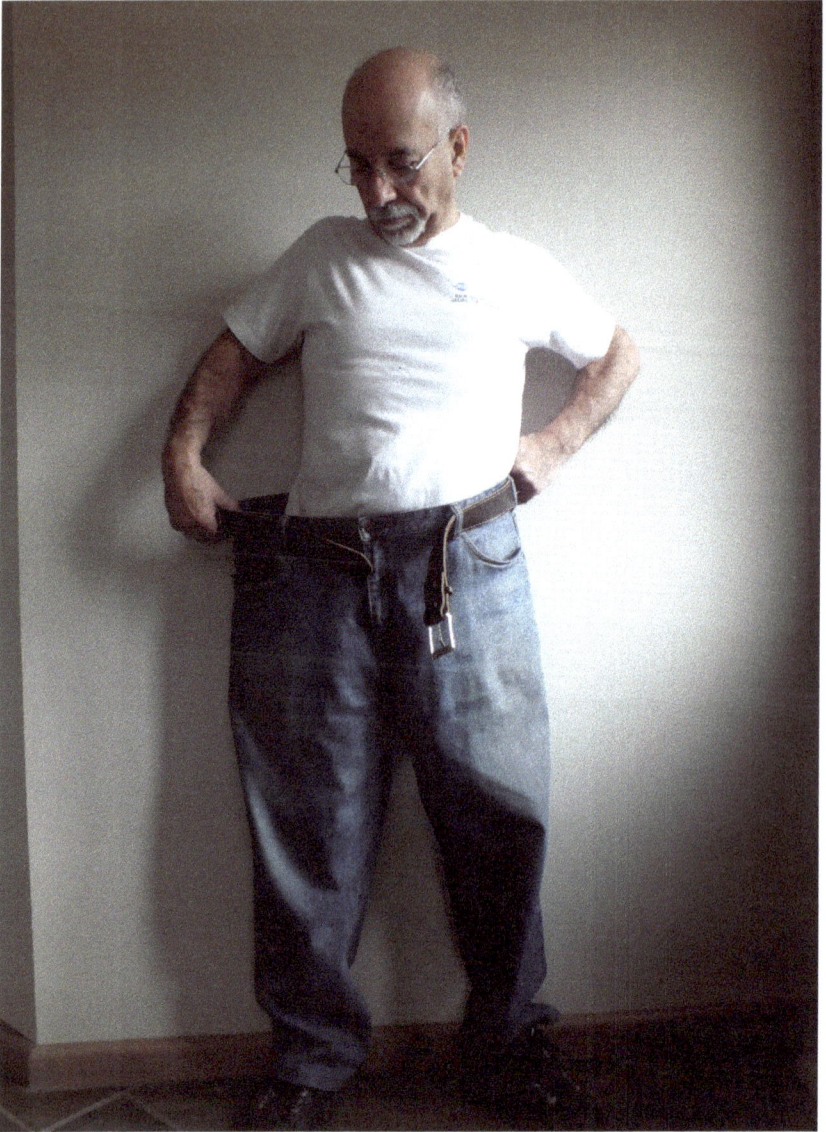

That's What Happens With Weight Loss.

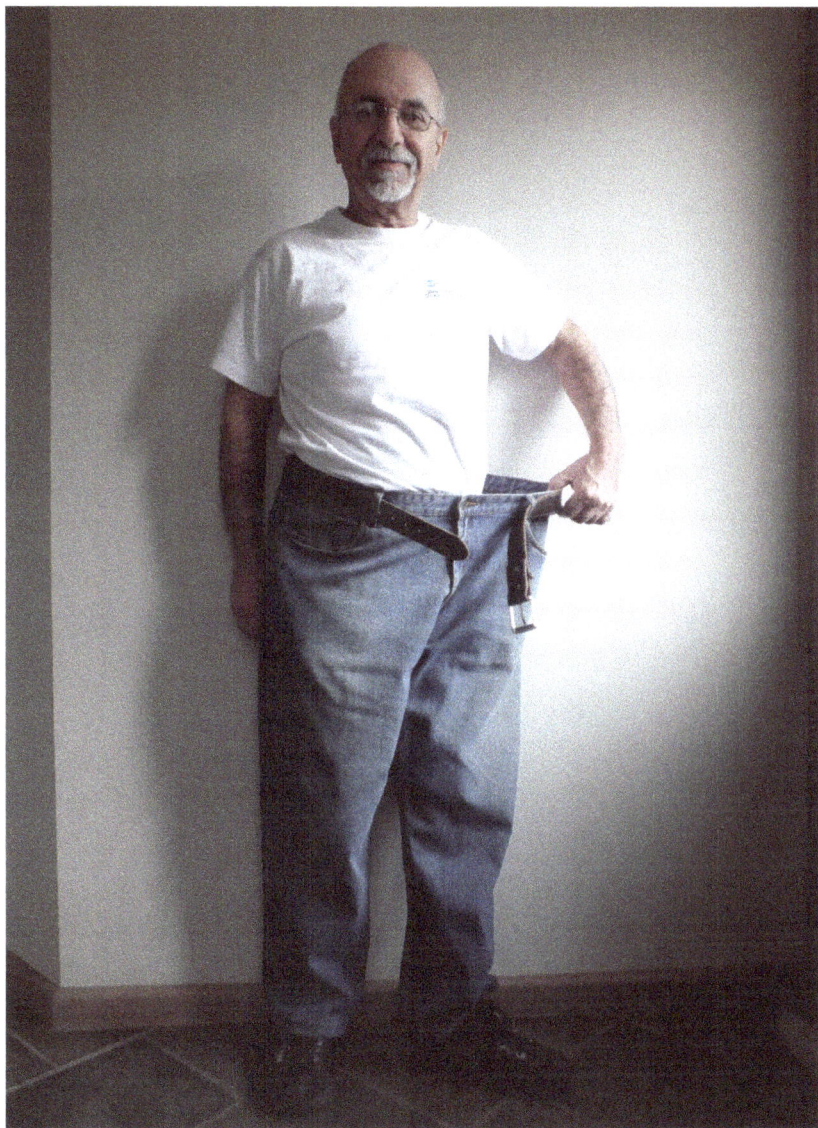

The New Me

Losing weight, a change of pace that I definitely do not regret taking.

So go forth with renewed energy knowing full well that you will win and successfully lose weight.

.

www.ingramcontent.com/pod-product-compliance
Lightning Source LLC
Chambersburg PA
CBHW051249020426
42333CB00025B/3131